THE NECESSITY OF DRINKING WATER

❧

BY PRISCILLA BRIGGETT BS RN BSN

ISBN 978-0-578-20159-7

Published by Visions Promotional Agency
Memphis, TN

Unless otherwise stated, Scripture is taken from the King James
Version Bible (KJV) which is public domain.

Cover and Interior Design by
Visions Promotional Agency
www.vpromoagency.com

Acknowledgements

I thank God for wisdom and knowledge to be a blessing to others. I thank my husband, Larry J., and my sons, Larry E., and Lance for listening, and all of your support. Evelyn Jones-Talley, thank you for encouraging and being a mentor to me as a nurse and a friend. Also, I would like to thank Breath of Life Christian Center and my Pastor and First Lady, Drs. Sammie and Addie Holloway, for your support, prayers, and allowing me to encourage members and others to drink water for a better lifestyle.

My prayer is that this information will encourage others to live a healthier life and be a blessing to their families and influence others to drink more water.

Kartriece Ward, LaShundra Starks and Elizabeth Hunter, thank you for making this a reality.

Table of Contents

Introduction

As I was preparing to teach at a women's conference, my prayer was, "How can I be a blessing to the women?" It came to me to teach on why water is needed and I titled it, "The Necessity of Water."

For the past few years, God has put on my heart to write a book about water. I was asked to present a teaching on water as it relates to your health. Most people would say things such as, "I don't drink much water because it doesn't taste like anything." and "Drinking a lot of water makes me go to the restroom, so....". The contents of this book will show you why drinking water is good for you. Hosea 4:6 tells it best, "My people are destroyed for lack of knowledge...". I hope the information presented will bless you, so that your life and health will never be the same.

❧

Isaiah 55:10 *"For as the rain cometh down, and the snow from heaven, and returneth not thither, but watereth the earth, and maketh it bring forth and bud, that it may give seed to the sower, and bread to the eater:"*

Water is LIFE!

What is Water?

By definition, water is a transparent, colorless, odorless, tasteless, liquid; a compound of hydrogen and oxygen, (H_2O), freezing at 32°F or 0°C, and boiling at 212°F or 100°C. [1,2]

A simple way to define water is the clear liquid that has no color, taste, or smell. It falls from clouds as rain and forms streams, lakes, and seas. It is also used for drinking, washing, and is the basis of the fluid of living organisms. [2]

ARE YOU DRINKING ENOUGH WATER???

Water Facts
Did You Know?

The human body is 50 to 75% water. An average adult can survive up to a month without food, but only 2 days to a week without water.

Other water facts are:

1. Lack of fluid causes dehydration.
2. Lack of fluid causes you to become tired.
3. Lack of fluid affects your concentration.
4. Lack of fluid affects your coordination.
5. Lack of fluid affects decision making skills.
6. Lack of fluid causes stress and depression.
7. The loss of fluid occurs continuously through sweat, urination, etc.
8. 71% percent of the earth's surface is made up of water. [13]

WATER in the human BODY ranges from **50-75%**

Life Without Water

Have you ever imagined how the world would be without water? Let's take a journey! Imagine taking a stroll to the neighborhood park. There is no grass, trees, lakes, or water fountains present. Only rocks, gravel, dirt, sand, and concrete. There are no birds, squirrels, turtles, or fish. The air is filled with dust, and trash has taken over the area. No children, dogs, cats or adults are present other than you and a homeless person sleeping on the park bench. The temperature is 99°F in July. The heat index is 112.

There is a heat advisory that will not expire for the next 72 hours. The heat wave started in mid- May. There is no water to be found. The residents who live in the city are moving away because there is a drought in the area. The neighborhood stores have been without water for several days, and there is no rain in sight. There are boarded houses and stores throughout the city. You can't take a bath, wash your belongings, or drink a glass of water. Can you imagine the future of the people who are living in that city? They need help!!

Now, imagine, two days later, the people prayed and it rained. Not only did it rain, it poured off and on for two days. On the third day, the sun shone brightly in the clear blue sky. The grass began to grow. The lakes, which were dried up, now contained water from the rain. The people started to move back into the city. The drought was over! Can you see how important the rain was to that city? Can you imagine how important water is for life?

Why Should I Drink Water?

As a registered nurse (RN), I often ask people, "When was the last time you drank some water?" Their responses vary. Some people would avoid answering the question, while others would say, "I know I need to drink more water." Good answer, but when? Some people would respond, "I keep water with me all the time," but I would never see them drinking it. The following are some very important reasons for you to drink water: [3, 9]

1. **WEIGHT LOSS** - Most people who drink water according to the suggestions of NIH (National Institute of Health) facts, lose weight.
2. **BOOSTS ENERGY** - When your body is hydrated, you will have more energy to perform different tasks.
3. **LOWER STRESS** - Drinking water daily will lower most stressors in your life (i.e. home, job, and vacation).
4. **BUILD MUSCLE TONE** - Drinking water aids in building muscle tone in your body.
5. **NOURISH YOUR SKIN** - When you drink water every day, your skin is tighter and healthier.
6. **DIGESTION** - Drinking water helps you to have a regular bowel movement, clean out your stomach, and assists in digestion of all the foods that we eat.

7. **INCREASES DECISION-MAKING SKILLS** – Drinking water hydrates your brain and helps you to think and make the right decisions.

8. **REDUCES KIDNEY STONES** – Drinking water aids in flushing out your urinary tract system thus decreasing formation of stones.

9. **REGULATES BODY TEMPERATURE** – Drinking water assists in lowering the body's temperature during hot and cold weather and when our bodies are sick (under attack).

10. **EYE HEALTH** – Drinking water hydrates your eyes and assists with clearer vision. [3, 9]

When your body is functioning abnormally, drinking water is a good resource to aid in correcting that problem. I am sure that you can add to this list. Think about how water makes a difference in our daily lives. Have you ever felt hot and sticky, and took a cool shower and felt better? Have you ever had a massage, and the person who did the massage encouraged you to drink water afterwards? Why is this? The cool shower assists in lowering your body's temperature, causing your body to be relaxed. Drinking water before and after a massage keeps your muscles from cramping. There are many benefits when you use and drink water every day.

Celebration One: Benefits

In nursing school, one of my professors used to tell us that every test is a celebration of the knowledge that we had learned. Each test was called a "celebration." This section of my book is a "celebration" of what you have learned about water. What are some very important reasons for you to drink water? [3, 9]

[Remember, celebration = test]

Write the letter in the blank that corresponds with the following items from 1 to 10.

1. LOSE WEIGHT ____

2. BOOSTS ENERGY ____

3. LOWER STRESS ____

4. BUILD MUSCLE TONE ____

5. NOURISH YOUR SKIN ____

6. DIGESTION ____

7. INCREASE DECISION MAKING SKILLS ____

8. REDUCES KIDNEY STONES ____

9. REGULATE BODY TEMPERATURE ____

10. EYE HEALTH ____

A. Drinking water hydrates our eyes and assists with clearer vision.

B. Aids in flushing out your urinary tract system and decreases formation of stones.

C. Drinking water helps you to have a regular bowel movement, clean out your stomach, and assists in the digestion of all foods that we eat each day.

D. Aids in building muscle tone in our body.

E. When your body is hydrated, you will have more energy to perform different tasks.

F. Most people who drink water, according to the suggestions of NIH facts, lose weight.

G. Drinking water daily will lower most stressors in your life (i.e. home, job, and vacation).

H. When you drink water every day, your skin is tighter and healthier.

I. Drinking water hydrates your brain, and helps you to think and make the right decisions.

J. Assists in lowering the body's temperature during hot and cold weather and when our bodies are sick (under attack).

Answers on page 36

How Can I Tell if I Am Not Drinking Enough Water?

Most people do not drink enough water on an average day. How do I know? Let's look at the six senses. You may be more familiar with the five senses. They are *sight, sound, touch, smell, and taste*. The sixth sense is *common* sense.

1. **Sight** - When your body is dehydrated, you can see a change in the color and elasticity of your skin. For example, someone may say that your skin looks pale.
2. **Sound** - Hearing is another way to tell if you are not drinking enough water. For example, you may hear your stomach growling. Your body is telling you to drink water. Listen to your body.
3. **Touch** - When you pinch, squeeze or pull on your skin, it will take a few seconds for it to fall back in place. Try it on yourself or someone you may be concerned about (with their permission of course).
4. **Smell** - Water has no smell; therefore, most people are not interested in it.
5. **Taste** - Dry mouth is a sign of not consuming enough water.
6. **Common Sense** - My definition of common sense is doing what you know is right.

Your body can be weak and frail when it is dehydrated. Your body can get dehydrated by the choices you make in life. For example: smoking, drinking alcoholic beverages or carbonated beverages, not eating the right foods, or eating too much food can also cause you to be dehydrated. How? These choices leave no room in your body for water. This is also where sickness and diseases come in. "Why do I have a headache?" "Why is my blood pressure so high?" Chances are your body is responding to a lack of hydration. When you feel thirsty, your body is already dehydrated. If your body feels weak or extra tired, you are probably dehydrated and need fluids in your body.

According to Hebrews 5:14, "But strong meat belongeth to them that are of full age, even those who by reason of use have their senses exercised to discern both good and evil." Using your six senses with discernment lets you know that drinking water is what God planned for you to have here on earth. Have you ever heard that water is life? Deuteronomy 30:15, 19, "See, I have set before thee this day life and good, and death and evil;" In verse 19, God tells us what to do: "I call heaven and earth to record this day against you, that I have set before you life and death, blessing and cursing: therefore choose life, that both thou and thy seed may live:" When you choose to drink water, you choose life. As a parent of two healthy boys, I encourage you to drink water and pass it on to your generations. [5]

Celebration Two: The Senses

This section is a "celebration" of what you have learned.

List the six senses to help you identify when you have not consumed enough water?
[Remember, celebration = test]

Fill in the blanks with the six senses.

1. _____

2. _____

3. _____

4. _____

5. _____

6. _____

Answers on page 36

LISTEN
to your body.

It will tell you,
"DRINK
more water!"

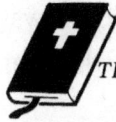

THE BIBLE SAYS...

What Does the Bible Say?

- 3 John 2 "Beloved, I wish above all things that thou mayest prosper and be in health, even as thy soul prospereth." [5]
    - God wants us to prosper and be in good health. The best way to prosper and be in good health is to drink more water. When your body is dehydrated or stressed, certain enzymes are destroyed. Enzymes are proteins that cause chemical reactions in our bodies that keep us alive, and in good health. [7]
- James 1:5 "If any of you lack wisdom, let him ask of God, that giveth to all men liberally, and upbraideth not; and it shall be given him."
    - If you lack wisdom, ask God for direction in all areas of your life. Drinking water is necessary and wise! Wisdom is better than gold. God loves us all. He said, if ANY man lack wisdom let him ask me [God] and I [God] will give it to him/her — no matter who you are, where you live, how much money you have, male or female, young or old. Remember, drinking water is wise!
- 2 Chronicles 7:14 "If my people, which are called by my name, shall humble themselves, and pray, and seek my

face, and turn from their wicked ways; then will I hear from heaven, and will forgive their sin, and will heal their land."

- In order for your land to be healed, something is required. You must do something in order to get results. This concept is important in every area of your life, especially health. The Bible tells us to seek God first! In addition, making an appointment to see a healthcare provider should be at the top of the list. Make sure you see someone who knows about your health history. For example, if you are a dialysis patient, your situation is different. Drinking too much water will negatively affect your health. The average person will benefit from drinking more water according to their lifestyle. It is very important to know what your body can and cannot handle. Do not get overwhelmed, as Matthew 6:33 tells us when we seek God he will give us the direction on what to do.

- Philippians 4:13 "I can do all things through Christ which strengtheneth me."
  Philippians 4:19 "But my God shall supply all your need according to his riches in glory by Christ Jesus." [5]

  - I have heard some people state, "It is not that I don't like water; I just don't want to drink water." Words are power packed! We have to watch what we say. Philippians 4:13 tells us Christ

Jesus gives us strength to do anything, even the things we do not want to do. God put water on the earth for us to utilize. I do not like mustard, but I make every effort to use mustard because of the health benefits of mustard. Drinking water has benefits.

Many illnesses can be resolved by what we eat and drink. Some examples are: asthma, hypertension, diabetes, and seasonal allergies. Think about how much money you could save by doing what is best for your health by drinking water every day!!

❧

(Selah.)
Pause & think about that!

The Costly Risk of Dehydration

According to WebMD, "An analysis of per capita health care spending in 2013 for people with diabetes found average costs were $14,999, around $10,000 higher than the average $4,305 in per capita spending." [10]

What does this mean to me? This means that most people would rather take medicine than drink water. You measure the cost. How much do you spend on medicine each month? Include prescriptions and over the counter medicine. I am not telling anyone not to take your medicine. In fact, ask your primary care doctor about drinking more water and your medical condition. If your health condition can tolerate drinking water, you will be healthier and save money.

As a registered nurse with medical surgical nursing experience, I have seen a lot of patients come in to be treated for dehydration. Most patients who are admitted are placed on IV fluids for two to three days before being discharged. This can be very costly for the patient. Dehydration can affect your health in ways that will negatively alter your every day life. When it is not dealt with at the root, this can escalate to major issues. I know from experience.

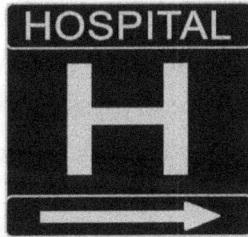

During my time of working 12-hour shifts (that can easily turn into 14 to 16 hours) in the hospital, I was so busy working and caring for patients, that I did not make time to drink water and eat regular meals. After working a 12-hour shift, I was tired, hungry, and dehydrated. I started to have chest pains. I called my primary healthcare doctor and made an appointment. When I said that I was having chest pains, they saw me right away. The nurse took my blood pressure and it was higher than normal. She stated that the last few times that I came in, my blood pressure had been high. The nurse and the doctor suggested that I start taking blood pressure medication. The doctor stated that I was stressed and dehydrated. I told the nurse practitioner, who then suggested that I change my diet. The doctor wrote me a prescription for blood pressure medication. I informed the doctor that I wanted to work on lowering my blood pressure without medication. He also wrote me a prescription for anxiety medication. I accepted the anxiety prescription, ordered the medication, yet did not take one pill.

I talked with a former RN coworker and she told me that she became addicted to the anxiety medication that her doctor gave her. It was the same medication that my doctor ordered for me. Instead of taking the medications, I started drinking water and I found a new job. When I went to have my annual physical, my blood pressure was normal! Glory to God! Decreased stress and increased intake of water improved my health.

Later, I was asked to do a health presentation at a women's conference. During my research, I read a book called; "*Water for Health, for Healing, for Life: You're not Sick, You're Thirsty!*" by F. Batmanghelidj M.D. In this book, Dr. Batmanghelidj talked about how he helped heal prisoners by drinking more water only and no use of medication. [8]

It was at that conference that God put on my heart to write my book. My goal is that this book will help other people to be healthier by drinking more water.

You're
NOT SICK
YOU are
THIRSTY

I have been taught that words are powerful. My pastor teaches and believes in speaking the Word of God. He teaches that faith without works, or action, is dead. I know for a fact that drinking water can -and has- made a difference in me and my family's life!

What Can I Do to Drink More Water?

So how much fluid does the average, healthy adult living in a temperate climate need? The National Academies of Sciences, Engineering, and Medicine determined that an adequate daily fluid intake is: [6]

- About 15.5 cups (3.7 liters) of fluids for men

- About 11.5 cups (2.7 liters) of fluids a day for women

These recommendations cover fluids from water, other beverages and food that we eat every day. About 20 percent of daily fluid intake usually comes from foods like fruits and vegetables and about 80 percent comes from drinking fluids. [4, 6]

The 2015-2020 Dietary Guidelines for Americans recommends that adults should eat 2 cups of fruit and 2.5 cups of vegetables per day. [4]

For example:

- The average adult male should drink 13 cups of water, and eat 2.5 cups of vegetables and/or 2 cups of fruits daily.
- The average adult female should drink 9 cups of water, and eat 2.5 cups of vegetables and/or 2 cups of fruits daily.

Note that the amount of fluid a person should drink per day is based on the person's activity level, health, where they live and the time of year. [4, 12]

Below I have given three suggestions on what you can do to drink more water every day.

SUGGESTION #1 – Consume the recommended number of cups of water.

Note: Every time you eat a meal, drink water for example:

Drinking Water Consumption Chart

= 8oz.	Wake-Up	Breakfast	Lunch	Snack	Dinner	Bedtime
MEN ♂	🥛🥛	🥛🥛🥛	🥛🥛	🥛🥛	🥛🥛	🥛🥛
Women ♀	🥛	🥛🥛	🥛🥛	🥛	🥛🥛	🥛

= 16.9 oz= 2 cups = 500mL

See page 37 for a Water Intake Form.

SUGGESTION #2 - Eat more fruits and vegetables. [4]

The Percent of Water in Fruits and Vegetables

Fruits % Water		Vegetables % Water	
	Watermelon 92%		Lettuce 96%
	Strawberries 92%		Cucumber 96%
	Grapefruit 91%	Zucchini 95%	
	Cantaloupe 90 %		Tomatoes (red) 94%
	Apple 84%	Carrots 87%	

SUGGESTION #3 – Plan your water consumption.

- Make drinking water available everywhere you go. Keep a bottle of water at your desk, in your bag, and at home.

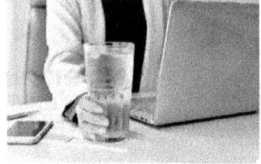

- Drink water or beverages that meet your needs. Try spring water or Gatorade, especially after you exercise or play sports.

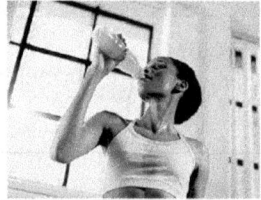

- Keep drinking water in a large container, (1 liter) and refill as often as needed. [11]

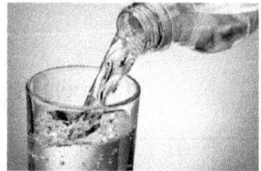

- Ask for drinking water instead of drinks, sodas, coffee or tea when you go out to eat. This can increase your water intake and save you money.

Summary and Review

- The National Institute of Health recommends 9 cups of water for women and 13 cups of water for men every day.
- There are many reasons that we should drink more water. Water promotes a better and healthier lifestyle! The bible states, "Beloved, I wish above all things that thou mayest prosper and be in health..." 3 John 1:2
- Water is natural and more than 75 percent of our body depends on it.
- We should drink water to lose weight, reduce stress, boost energy, hydrate our joints, increase vision, ease hunger pains, and lower our blood pressure. [4]
- Do not over medicate when you can drink water and be hydrated.
- Three ways to drink more water are: drink with meals, eat more fruits and vegetables, and make water available.

Drink Water!

When my sons were young boys, they played soccer during the summer at the church that we attend. Their coach's name was Mark. At every practice and at each game, Coach Mark made sure the teams had plenty of water to drink. Drinking water made a difference in how they played on the soccer field. Regardless of the time of year, practice keeping water available.

The necessity of drinking water is for life. Our bodies can dry up just like the city that was dying due to lack of water. The word of God says that our body is our temple. We need to take care of it in order to live a healthier and more productive life. When you drink water, you can enjoy the life that God created for you, be a blessing to yourself and to those around you. Start by asking yourself, "Have I had any water today?"

THE END

REFERENCES

1. http://www.dictionary.com/browse/water

2. https://www.merriam.webster.com/dictionary/water

3. http://www.healthbenefit-of-water.com/benefit-of-drinking-water.html

4. https://healthyeating.sfgate.com/list-fruits-vegetable-high-water-content-8958.html

5. King James Version, All scripture references.

6. Mayo Clinic Staff. (2017, September 6). *Water: How much should you drink every day?*. Retrieved from https://www.mayoclinic.org/healthy-lifestyle/nutrition-and-healthy-eating/in-depth/water/art-20044256

7. Newman. Tim. (2018, January 11) https://www.medicalnewstoday.com/articles/319704

8. *Water for Health, for Healing, for Life: You're not Sick, You're Thirsty!*; F. *Batmanghelidj. M.D.* June 2003 pg 26

9. Zelman. K. M. (2008, May 8). *6 Reasons to Drink Water.* Retrieved from https://www.webmd.com/diet/features/6-reasons-to-drink-water

10. Andrews, M. (2017). *Diabetes Drug Costs Overlooked, But Shouldn't Be.* Retrieved from https://www.webmd.com/health-insurance/news/20150818/cost-of-diabetes-drugs-often-overlooked-but-it-shouldnt-be#1

11. www.istockphoto.com

12. Marcin, A. (2017, April 19). *How Much Water You Need to Drink.* Retrieved from https://www.healthline.com/health/how-much-water-should-I-drink#recommendations

13. Bartel, A. (2018, February 4). *50 Amazing Water Facts That Everyone Should Know.* Retrieved from https://iwaterpurification.com/water-facts/

DISCLAIMER

- Check with your primary care doctor before starting anything new.
- Certain medical or physical conditions will not allow you to drink large amounts of water.
- Please use this and all information with caution when it comes to your health.

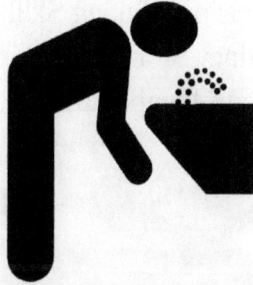

DRINK MORE WATER!!

CELEBRATION ANSWERS

Celebration One: Benefits

1. Lose Weight   F
2. Boosts Energy   E
3. Lower Stress   G
4. Build Muscle Tone   D
5. Nourish Your Skin   H
6. Digestion   C
7. Increase Decision-Making Skills   I
8. Reduces Kidney Stones   B
9. Regulate Body Temperature   J
10. Eye Health   A

Celebration Two: The Senses

1. Sight
2. Sound
3. Touch
4. Smell
5. Taste
6. Common Sense

Water Intake Form

Follow these three steps and use this form to assist in reaching your daily water goal for a healthier lifestyle.

STEP 1: Set an obtainable goal.

Example - My goal is 3 cups of water daily for one week. I will drink one cup in the morning, one cup at noon day and one cup at night to assist in monitoring my water intake for a healthier lifestyle. Week two increase your goal to 3-6 cups daily.

STEP 2: Keep water accessible for easier consumption.

STEP 3: Monitor your daily water intake. Within the chart mark a line for each cup of water you consume. Mark two lines for each 16.9 oz. bottle of water you consume. Tally your total at the end of each day.

| = 1 cup || = 16.9 oz bottle of water

Week of: _____   My Daily Goal = _____ cups

	Morning 6:00 AM – 11:59 AM	Afternoon 12:00 PM – 6:59 PM	Night 7:00 PM – 11:59 PM	TOTAL (Daily Total)
Sunday				
Monday				
Tuesday				
Wednesday				
Thursday				
Friday				
Saturday				

THE REAL CELEBRATION IS GOOD HEALTH!

A HEALTHY LIFE AND A HEALTHY LIFESTYLE MAKE A HEALTHIER YOU!

START BY ASKING YOURSELF, "HAVE I HAD ANY WATER TODAY?"

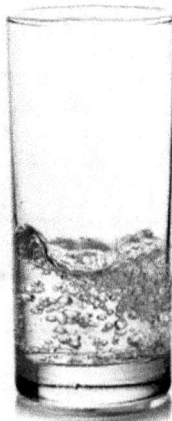

About the Author

Priscilla Briggett is a wife and mother of two boys. She resides in TN and is a RN BSN, Transitional Care Nurse/Case Manager, and a certified CPR Instructor. For over 25 years she has had a heart for seeing others healthy.

To contact the author email, DrinkH2O@yahoo.com. All testimonials, suggestions and comments are welcome.

NOTES

NOTES